Focus Forward:

Navigating Life with Attention
Deficit Hyperactivity Disorder
(ADHD)

Mark Winters

Focus Forward: Navigating Life with Attention Deficit
Hyperactivity Disorder (ADHD)
Author Mark Winters
© 2024 Neil McKenzie. All Rights Reserved
Published By Neil McKenzie
ISBN 9781445231709
Imprint: Lulu.com

Focus Forward: Navigating Life with attention deficit hyperactivity disorder
(ADHD)

Introduction:

Coping as an adult or Child diagnosed with ADHD.

The struggles with focus, organisation, and impulsivity.

Diagnosis and Denial:

Receiving a diagnosis of ADHD, but initially struggling to accept it.

Facing stigma and misunderstanding from family, friends, and peers.

Seeking Support:

Seeking guidance from a therapist specialising in ADHD.

Through therapy sessions, beginning to understand their condition and develop coping strategies.

Embracing Differences:

Embracing the unique strengths and talents associated with ADHD. - Discovering that creativity, hyperfocus, and spontaneity can be assets in certain situations.

Navigating Education:

Facing challenges in academic settings due to ADHD symptoms. - Getting support from educators and accommodations and learn to excel in school.

Managing Relationships:

Struggling with maintaining friendships and romantic relationships. - Working on communication skills and boundaries to foster healthy connections.

Career Exploration:

Entering the workforce and encountering difficulties in finding and maintaining employment.

With career counselling and workplace accommodations, discovering fulfilling career paths that align with the strengths.

Overcoming Obstacles:

Despite progress, facing setbacks and obstacles along the way. - Experiencing periods of frustration and self-doubt but persevere through resilience and determination.

Building a Support Network:

Finding support and camaraderie in ADHD support groups and communities.

Forming meaningful connections with others who share similar experiences and challenges.

Advocacy and Empowerment:

Inspired by the journey, becoming an advocate for ADHD awareness and acceptance.

Sharing your story publicly, advocating for improved resources and support for individuals with ADHD.

Finding Balance:

Striking a balance between managing their ADHD symptoms and embracing your true self.

Prioritising self-care, mindfulness, and healthy habits to maintain overall well-being.

Reflection and Growth:

Reflecting on the journey of coping with ADHD and the lessons learned along the way.

Celebrating the achievements and acknowledge the progress made in embracing your identity.

Introduction:

- Coping as an adult or Child diagnosed with ADHD.

 - The struggles with focus, organisation, and impulsivity.

Coping Strategies for Adults and Children Diagnosed with ADHD

Living with Attention Deficit Hyperactivity Disorder (ADHD) presents unique challenges, both for children and adults. The journey can be akin to navigating rapids —full of twists, turns, and occasional turbulence. However, with the right strategies and support systems in place, individuals diagnosed with ADHD can steer their way to calmer waters and lead fulfilling lives.

Understanding ADHD:

ADHD is a neurodevelopmental disorder characterised by difficulties with attention, hyperactivity, and impulsivity. While commonly diagnosed in childhood, many individuals carry the challenges of ADHD into adulthood, where they can manifest in various ways, impacting work, relationships, and overall well-being.

Coping Strategies for Children with ADHD:

1. Structured Environment:
Establishing routines and clear expectations can provide stability and predictability, which are beneficial for children with ADHD.

Utilise visual aids, such as charts and calendars, to help organise tasks and activities.

2. Positive Reinforcement:

Encourage and reward positive behaviour to reinforce desired actions.

Break tasks into manageable steps and celebrate accomplishments along the way.

3. Effective Communication:

Maintain open communication with teachers and caregivers to ensure consistency in support and intervention strategies.

Teach children to advocate for themselves and express their needs effectively.

4. Physical Outlets:

Engage children in regular physical activity to help channel excess energy in a constructive manner.

Explore hobbies and activities that align with their interests and strengths.

Coping Strategies for Adults with ADHD:

1. Time Management Techniques:
Use tools such as planners, digital calendars, and reminders to stay organised and manage deadlines effectively.

Break tasks into smaller, manageable chunks to prevent overwhelm.

2. Mindfulness and Meditation:

Practice mindfulness exercises to enhance focus and reduce impulsivity.

Incorporate relaxation techniques, such as deep breathing and progressive muscle relaxation, to manage stress and anxiety.

3. Seeking Support:

Build a strong support network of friends, family, and
healthcare professionals who understand

ADHD and can provide encouragement and guidance.
Consider joining support groups or online communities to
connect with others facing similar challenges.

4. Career Strategies: Identify career paths and
environments that align with strengths and interests,
allowing for greater engagement and job satisfaction.

Communicate with employers about ADHD-related
accommodations, such as flexible work arrangements
or assistive technologies.

Embracing Neurodiversity:

ADHD is not a character flaw or a sign of incompetence; it is a neurodevelopmental difference that comes with both challenges and strengths. By embracing neurodiversity, individuals with ADHD can recognise and harness their unique talents, creativity, and resilience to thrive in a world that may not always understand them.

Living with ADHD presents its share of rapids and obstacles, but with resilience, self-awareness, and support, individuals diagnosed with ADHD can navigate these challenges and emerge stronger on the other side. By implementing coping strategies tailored to their needs and embracing their neurodiversity, they can chart a course towards success, fulfilment, and wellbeing in all aspects of life.

Remember, the journey with ADHD is not about conquering the rapids but learning to navigate them with courage, resilience, and grace. You are not alone, and with each twist and turn, you grow stronger, more

resilient, and more capable of charting your path to success. [OBJ]

The Struggles of Focus, Organisation, and Impulsivity in ADHD

Attention Deficit Hyperactivity Disorder (ADHD) is more than just a diagnosis; it's a daily journey marked by struggles with focus, organisation, and impulsivity. Whether diagnosed in childhood or adulthood, individuals with ADHD often find themselves navigating through a maze of challenges that can affect every aspect of their lives.

The Battle with Focus:

One of the hallmark symptoms of ADHD is difficulty with sustained attention. For children, this may manifest as an inability to stay on task, frequent daydreaming, or easily getting sidetracked during activities. Adults with ADHD may struggle to concentrate on work tasks, often jumping from one task to another without completing them. The constant battle to maintain focus can lead to feelings of frustration, inadequacy, and self-doubt.

Organisational Hurdles:

Organisation is another area where individuals with ADHD often face significant obstacles. For children, this might mean forgetting homework assignments, losing school materials, or having a disorganised backpack. Adults with ADHD may struggle with managing finances, keeping track of appointments, or maintaining a tidy living or workspace. The chaos caused by organisational challenges can create stress, overwhelm, and feelings of being overwhelmed.

Impulsivity:

Impulsivity is a common trait in ADHD, characterised by acting without considering the consequences. Children with ADHD may blurt out answers in class, interrupt others during conversations, or engage in risky behaviours without thinking ahead. Adults with ADHD may struggle with impulsive spending, making decisions without fully considering the ramifications, or speaking before thinking. The impulsivity associated with ADHD can lead to social difficulties, strained relationships, and regrets.

Navigating Daily Life:

Living with ADHD means constantly navigating through a world that may not always understand or accommodate its challenges. Simple tasks that others take for granted—like following a conversation, completing a project, or remembering appointments—can feel like insurmountable hurdles. The relentless struggle to stay focused, organised, and in control can take a toll on self-esteem, mental health, and overall well-being.

Coping Strategies:

Despite the challenges, there is hope for individuals with ADHD. With the right support, strategies, and interventions, it's possible to manage symptoms and lead a fulfilling life. Some coping strategies include:

1. Medication: For many individuals with ADHD, medication can help improve focus, concentration, and impulse control.

2. Therapy: Cognitive-behavioural therapy (CBT) and other forms of therapy can teach coping skills, organisational strategies, and emotional regulation techniques.

3. Lifestyle Changes: Regular exercise, healthy eating habits, and adequate sleep can positively impact ADHD symptoms.

4. Support Systems: Building a strong support network of friends, family, and healthcare professionals who

understand ADHD can provide invaluable support and encouragement. Living with ADHD is a daily struggle marked by challenges with focus, organisation, and impulsivity. However, with understanding, support, and effective coping strategies, individuals with ADHD can navigate through life's maze and unlock their full potential. It's a journey marked by resilience, determination, and the courage to keep moving forward despite the obstacles.

Remember, ADHD does not define you. It's just one aspect of who you are—a unique individual with strengths, talents, and limitless potential. Embrace your journey, seek support when needed, and never underestimate the power of resilience in overcoming life's challenges. [OBJ]

2. Diagnosis and Denial:

 - Receiving a diagnosis of ADHD, but initially struggling to accept it.

- Facing stigma and misunderstanding from family, friends, and peers.

Receiving Diagnosis but Initially Struggling to Accept It

Receiving a diagnosis of attention deficit hyperactivity disorder (ADHD) can be a watershed moment in one's life. For many, it's a revelation that explains years of struggles with focus, organisation, and impulsivity. However, for others, the diagnosis may initially provoke feelings of denial, confusion, and even resistance. This journey of acceptance is not always linear but is marked by introspection, self-discovery, and ultimately, embracing the unseen aspects of oneself. Denial and Disbelief:

Upon first hearing the diagnosis, it's not uncommon to experience a sense of disbelief. Questions swirl in the mind—how could this label apply to me? Surely, it must be a mistake or an overreaction. Denial may lead to a refusal to acknowledge the validity of the diagnosis, dismissing it as a passing phase or a misinterpretation of normal behaviour.

Fear and Uncertainty:

Beneath the surface of denial often lies a deeper fear and uncertainty. Fear of the unknown—what does this diagnosis mean for my future? Will it limit my opportunities or define my identity? Uncertainty about how to navigate through life with ADHD—how do I manage symptoms, cope with challenges, and find acceptance in a world that may not fully understand?

Navigating Stigma and Shame:

Stigma and shame can also accompany an ADHD diagnosis, fuelled by misconceptions and societal judgments. Internalised beliefs that ADHD is a character flaw, or a sign of weakness may lead to feelings of inadequacy and self-doubt. The fear of being judged or misunderstood by others can create barriers to seeking support and embracing one's true self.

The Journey to Acceptance:

Despite the initial struggles, the journey towards acceptance of an ADHD diagnosis is marked by moments of introspection, self-awareness, and growth. It begins with a willingness to confront and challenge preconceived notions and societal stereotypes. It involves seeking knowledge and understanding about ADHD, its symptoms, and its impact on daily life.

Breaking Free from Labels:

Acceptance of an ADHD diagnosis is not about being defined by a label, but rather, recognising it as a part of oneself—a unique aspect that contributes to one's strengths, challenges, and experiences. It's about reframing perceptions and embracing neurodiversity—a celebration of the diverse ways in which our brains are wired.

Embracing Support and Resources:

Seeking support from loved ones, healthcare professionals, and peer communities can play a pivotal role in the journey towards acceptance. Therapy, counselling, and support groups provide safe spaces for validation, empathy, and shared experiences. Education about ADHD and learning effective coping strategies empower individuals to navigate through life's challenges with resilience and confidence.

Receiving a diagnosis of ADHD and struggling to accept it is a deeply personal journey—one marked by denial, fear, and uncertainty. Yet, through introspection, education, and support, individuals can embark on a path towards acceptance, self-discovery, and empowerment. It's a journey of embracing the unseen aspects of oneself, breaking free from labels, and celebrating the unique strengths and perspectives that ADHD brings.

Remember, acceptance is not about erasing the challenges of ADHD but rather, embracing them as integral parts of your journey. It's about finding strength in vulnerability, courage in self-awareness, and resilience in the face of adversity. In accepting your ADHD diagnosis, you pave the way for greater self-understanding, self-compassion, and ultimately, a life lived authentically and fully.

Facing Stigma and Misunderstanding from Family, Friends and Peers

Living with Attention Deficit Hyperactivity Disorder (ADHD) can often feel like a journey through a landscape marked by not only personal struggles but also societal perceptions. Stigma and misunderstanding from family, friends, and peers can compound the challenges faced by individuals with ADHD, creating barriers to acceptance, support, and understanding.

The Weight of Misconceptions:

From an early age, individuals with ADHD may encounter misconceptions and stereotypes perpetuated by society. ADHD is often misunderstood as a mere lack of discipline or laziness, rather than a neurodevelopmental disorder rooted in differences in brain function. These misconceptions can lead to judgments, criticism, and a sense of being unfairly labelled.

Family Dynamics:

Within the family unit, misunderstandings about ADHD can strain relationships and communication. Well-meaning parents may misinterpret symptoms of ADHD as defiance or disobedience, leading to disciplinary measures that exacerbate feelings of shame and inadequacy in the individual. Siblings may feel resentment or frustration towards the extra attention or accommodations given to the individual with ADHD, further perpetuating tensions within the family dynamic.

Challenges Among Peers:

Among peers, individuals with ADHD may face ridicule, ostracisation, or bullying due to differences in behaviour or social interactions. Difficulty with impulse control or social cues can lead to misunderstandings or misinterpretations of intentions, making it challenging to form meaningful connections or friendships. The fear of rejection or judgment may lead individuals with ADHD to mask their struggles, further isolating them from social support networks.

Navigating Friendship Circles:

Even within friendship circles, stigma and misunderstanding can rear their heads. Peers may perceive individuals with ADHD as unreliable, forgetful, or irresponsible, leading to exclusion from social activities or group projects. Well-intentioned advice to "just focus" or "try harder" overlooks the neurobiological factors underlying ADHD and undermines the individual's struggles and efforts to cope with their symptoms.

Overcoming Stigma and Building Understanding:

Breaking down stigma and fostering understanding begins with education and awareness. Providing accurate information about ADHD—its symptoms, challenges, and treatments—can dispel misconceptions and promote empathy and support. Encouraging open dialogue and communication within families and social circles creates opportunities for mutual understanding and acceptance.

Seeking Support and Advocacy:

Individuals with ADHD can find strength in seeking support from advocacy groups, mental health professionals, and peer communities. Connecting with others who share similar experiences fosters a sense of belonging and validation, reducing feelings of isolation and shame. Advocating for accommodations and support services in academic, work, and social settings empowers individuals with ADHD to thrive and succeed on their own terms.

Facing stigma and misunderstanding from family, friends, and peers can add layers of complexity to the already challenging journey of living with ADHD. However, by promoting education, fostering empathy, and advocating for support and understanding, individuals with ADHD can navigate through societal perceptions and cultivate environments that embrace their unique strengths and perspectives.

Remember, you are more than the label of ADHD. Your struggles do not define you, but your resilience, courage, and determination to overcome them do. By standing tall in the face of stigma and misunderstanding, you pave the way for greater awareness, acceptance, and inclusivity for all individuals living with ADHD.

3. Seeking Support:

 - Seeking guidance from a therapist specialising in ADHD.

- Through therapy sessions, beginning to understand their condition and develop coping strategies

Seeking Guidance from a Therapist Specialising In ADHD

In the labyrinth of life, some paths are more convoluted than others, and for those navigating the intricacies of attention deficit hyperactivity disorder (ADHD), the journey can often feel like charting a course through a stormy sea. Amidst the whirlwind of thoughts, emotions, and impulses, seeking guidance becomes not just an option but a beacon of hope, illuminating the way towards understanding and managing ADHD.

For many individuals grappling with ADHD, the decision to seek assistance from a therapist specialising in this neurodevelopmental disorder can mark a pivotal moment of empowerment. It's an acknowledgment that while ADHD may present its unique challenges, it doesn't define one's entirety nor dictate their destiny. Instead, it's an invitation to explore strategies, gain insights, and cultivate resilience under the guidance of a compassionate professional.

The journey begins with a simple yet profound step: reaching out. In a world often shrouded in stigma surrounding mental health, this act of vulnerability transforms into an act of courage. Whether it's scheduling that first appointment or mustering the courage to open up about one's struggles, each step forward is a testament to resilience and a commitment to self-growth.

Walking into the therapist's office, there's a palpable sense of relief—a sanctuary where judgment gives way to understanding, and silence yields to validation. Here, the therapist serves as more than a mere guide; they become a trusted confidant, a collaborator in unraveling the complexities of ADHD. Through active listening and empathetic presence, they create a safe space where thoughts can flow freely, unencumbered by fear or shame.

In the realm of ADHD therapy, one size certainly does not fit all. Therapists specialising in ADHD recognise the heterogeneous nature of the disorder, tailoring their approach to suit each individual's unique needs and circumstances. From behavioural techniques to mindfulness practices, the therapeutic toolbox brims with an array of strategies aimed at fostering self-awareness and building coping skills.

Central to this therapeutic journey is psychoeducation— an opportunity to demystify ADHD and shed light on its multifaceted nature. By understanding the underlying mechanisms of the disorder —ranging from executive dysfunction to emotional dysregulation—individuals gain a sense of agency, no longer held captive by misconceptions or self-doubt. Instead, they become active participants in their own healing, armed with knowledge and equipped with resilience.

Yet, therapy extends far beyond the confines of the therapist's office; it permeates every facet of life, influencing how one perceives oneself and interacts with the world. Through exploration and experimentation, individuals with ADHD learn to harness their strengths and navigate their challenges with newfound clarity and confidence. From creating structured routines to practicing mindfulness, each small victory serves as a testament to the transformative power of therapy.

Amidst the ebb and flow of progress, setbacks inevitably arise—a missed deadline, a forgotten appointment, a moment of impulsivity. Yet, within the therapeutic journey, setbacks are not met with condemnation but with compassion—a reminder that growth is nonlinear, and resilience lies in resilience.

As the therapeutic journey unfolds, individuals with ADHD begin to rewrite their narrative—not as victims of circumstance but as champions of resilience, navigating the turbulent waters of ADHD with grace and tenacity. With each passing session, they emerge not unscathed but strengthened, embracing their journey with newfound courage and unwavering determination.

In the embrace of a therapist's guidance, individuals with ADHD discover that their journey is not a solitary one but a shared odyssey—one marked by empathy, understanding, and the unwavering belief that, with the right support, even the most turbulent seas can be navigated.

Through Therapy Sessions, Beginning to Understand Their Condition and Develop Coping Strategies

Therapy becomes not just a sanctuary but a crucible for transformation—a space where understanding blooms and coping strategies take root in individuals grappling with attention deficit hyperactivity disorder (ADHD)

The journey begins with a simple yet profound question: What is ADHD? Through the lens of psycho-education, individuals embark on a voyage of discovery, unpacking the intricacies of their neurodevelopmental condition. From the hallmark symptoms of inattention and impulsivity to the lesser-known nuances of executive dysfunction, each revelation serves as a beacon of illumination, dispelling the shadows of confusion and self-doubt.

As understanding blossoms, so too does self-compassion —a tender acknowledgment that ADHD is not a flaw to be fixed but a facet of one's identity to be embraced. In the gentle embrace of therapy, individuals with ADHD learn to rewrite their narrative, no longer defined by their struggles but empowered by their resilience. Through empathy and validation, the therapist becomes not just a guide but a partner in this journey of self-discovery—a witness to the unfolding of potential.

Yet, understanding alone is not enough; it is but the first step in a broader quest for mastery. Armed with insights gleaned from therapy sessions, individuals begin to cultivate coping strategies—tools to navigate the ebbs and flows of ADHD with grace and resilience. From time management techniques to organisational skills, the therapeutic toolbox brims with an array of strategies tailored to suit each individual's unique needs and circumstances.

Central to this process is the cultivation of self-awareness—a deepening understanding of one's strengths, weaknesses, and triggers. Through reflection and introspection, individuals learn to recognise the patterns and pitfalls of their ADHD, transforming moments of frustration into opportunities for growth. With each passing session, they emerge not just as survivors but as architects of their own destiny—empowered by the knowledge that, with the right support, even the most daunting challenges can be surmounted.

Yet, therapy extends far beyond the confines of the therapist's office; it permeates every facet of life, influencing how one perceives oneself and interacts with the world. From the structured routines of daily life to the mindful cultivation of resilience, coping strategies become not just a means of managing ADHD but a way of life—a testament to the transformative power of therapy.

In the crucible of therapy, individuals with ADHD discover that their journey is not a solitary one but a shared odyssey—one marked by empathy, understanding, and the unwavering belief that, with the right support, anything is possible. Through therapy, they unlock the door to their true potential, stepping boldly into a future filled with promise and possibility.

4. Embracing Differences:

- Embracing the unique strengths and talents associated with ADHD.

- Discovering that creativity, hyperfocus, and spontaneity can be assets in certain situations

Embracing their unique strengths and talents associated with ADHD

In a world often fixated on conformity, the notion of celebrating neurodiversity can seem like a radical concept. Yet, within the tapestry of human experience, there exists a kaleidoscope of minds—each one bearing its unique hue, its distinctive brilliance. For individuals navigating the labyrinth of attention deficit hyperactivity disorder (ADHD), this brilliance often lies dormant, obscured by the shadows of stigma and misconception. But within the gentle embrace of therapy, a revelation unfolds—a recognition that ADHD is not merely a collection of deficits but a mosaic of strengths waiting to be unveiled.

At the heart of this revelation lies a simple yet profound truth: ADHD is not a monolith but a spectrum—a spectrum teeming with creativity, resilience, and boundless energy. From the whirlwind of thoughts that spark innovation to the unbridled passion that fuels creativity, the hallmarks of ADHD are not just challenges to be overcome but gifts to be celebrated.

In the quiet confines of the therapist's office, individuals with ADHD embark on a journey of self-discovery—a journey marked by introspection, revelation, and empowerment. Through the lens of psychoeducation, they come to understand the intricate interplay of their neurobiology—the ebbs and flows of attention, the dance of impulsivity, the symphony of hyperactivity. But amidst the cacophony of symptoms lies a hidden treasure trove —a reservoir of untapped potential waiting to be unleashed.

As therapy unfolds, individuals begin to peel back the layers of self-doubt and insecurity, revealing the brilliance that lies beneath. From the depths of their struggles emerges a newfound sense of self-awareness—a recognition of their unique strengths and talents. Whether it's the ability to hyperfocus on tasks of passion, the capacity to think outside the box, or the talent for multitasking in high-pressure environments, each revelation serves as a testament to the inherent gifts of ADHD.

Yet, embracing these strengths is not without its challenges. In a world that often values conformity over creativity, individuals with ADHD may find themselves marginalized or misunderstood. But within the sanctuary of therapy, they find solace—a safe space where their brilliance is not just acknowledged but celebrated. Through validation and empowerment, they learn to stand tall in their uniqueness, unapologetically embracing the gifts that set them apart.

Beyond the confines of therapy, the journey of self-discovery continues—a journey marked by resilience, courage, and unwavering determination. Armed with the knowledge that their ADHD is not a limitation but a source of strength, individuals begin to navigate the world with newfound confidence and purpose. From the boardroom to the classroom, from the studio to the stage, they leave an indelible mark—a testament to the transformative power of embracing one's true self.

In the embrace of therapy, individuals with ADHD discover that their brilliance is not a burden but a blessing—a beacon of light illuminating the path towards self-acceptance and fulfilment. With each passing day, they step boldly into the world, their hearts ablaze with the knowledge that they are not just surviving with ADHD—they are thriving, empowered by their unique gifts and talents.

Discovering that creativity, hyperfocus, and spontaneity can be assets in certain situations

In the grand tapestry of human experience, diversity reigns supreme—a symphony of minds, each imbued with its unique rhythm, its distinctive melody. Yet, amidst the cacophony of existence, there exists a subset of minds whose brilliance often defies convention. For individuals navigating the maze of attention deficit hyperactivity disorder (ADHD), this brilliance often lies dormant, obscured by the shadows of stigma and misconception. But within the gentle embrace of therapy, a revelation unfolds—a recognition that what society perceives as deficits can, in fact, be powerful assets.

At the heart of this revelation lies a simple yet profound truth: ADHD is not a limitation but a lens— a lens through which the world is perceived with unparalleled clarity and intensity. From the chaos of thoughts that spark innovation to the laser-like focus that propels productivity, the hallmarks of ADHD are not just challenges to be overcome but gifts to be celebrated.

In the sanctuary of therapy, individuals with ADHD embark on a journey of self-discovery—a journey marked by introspection, revelation, and empowerment. Through the lens of psychoeducation, they come to understand the intricate interplay of their neurobiology—the ebb and flow of attention, the dance of impulsivity, the symphony of hyperactivity. But amidst the chaos lies a hidden treasure trove—a reservoir of untapped potential waiting to be unleashed.

As therapy unfolds, individuals begin to peel back the layers of self-doubt and insecurity, revealing the brilliance that lies beneath. From the depths of their struggles emerge a newfound sense of self-awareness—a recognition of their unique strengths and talents. Whether it's the ability to think outside the box, the capacity for hyperfocus on tasks of passion, or the talent for spontaneous creativity, each revelation serves as a testament to the inherent gifts of ADHD.

Creativity, once seen as a flight of fancy, emerges as a formidable asset—a wellspring of innovation and inspiration. In the studio, the classroom, or the boardroom, individuals with ADHD breathe life into ideas that defy convention, reshaping the world with their unique vision.

Hyperfocus, once dismissed as a fleeting distraction, becomes a superpower—a laser-like focus that propels productivity and drives success. In the midst of chaos, individuals with ADHD immerse themselves in tasks of passion, harnessing their boundless energy to achieve feats that defy expectation.

Spontaneity, once feared as a liability, emerges as a catalyst for adventure—a willingness to embrace the unknown and seize the moment. From impromptu adventures to last-minute solutions, individuals with ADHD navigate life with a sense of spontaneity that infuses each day with excitement and possibility.

Yet, embracing these assets is not without its challenges. In a world that often values conformity over creativity, individuals with ADHD may find themselves marginalised or misunderstood. But within the sanctuary of therapy, they find solace—a safe space where their brilliance is not just acknowledged but celebrated. Through validation and empowerment, they learn to stand tall in their uniqueness, unapologetically embracing the gifts that set them apart.

In the embrace of therapy, individuals with ADHD discover that their brilliance is not a burden but a blessing —a beacon of light illuminating the path towards self-acceptance and fulfilment. With each passing day, they step boldly into the world, their hearts ablaze with the knowledge that they are not just surviving with ADHD— they are thriving, empowered by their unique gifts and talents.

5. Navigating Education:

- Facing challenges in academic settings due to ADHD symptoms.

- Getting support from educators and accommodations and learn to excel in school.

Facing Challenges in Academic Settings Due to ADHD Symptoms

Navigating the academic terrain is often a labyrinth of challenges for many students, but for those grappling with attention deficit hyperactivity disorder (ADHD), the journey can feel like traversing through a dense fog. ADHD, characterised by difficulties in concentration, impulse control, and hyperactivity, casts its shadow over every facet of life, including academia. For these students, the classroom becomes a battleground where traditional learning structures often clash with their unique cognitive makeup, leaving them feeling overwhelmed and misunderstood.

One of the hallmark symptoms of ADHD is an inability to sustain attention for extended periods, making it arduous for students to stay focused during lectures or while reading textbooks. The mere act of sitting still and absorbing information becomes an uphill struggle, as their minds dart from one thought to another like a pinball machine in overdrive. Consequently, crucial details may slip through the cracks, leaving them perpetually playing catch-up in their studies.

Furthermore, the executive function impairments associated with ADHD can wreak havoc on organisational skills and time management. Assignments pile up like a mountain, and deadlines loom ominously overhead, yet the ability to prioritise tasks and manage time effectively remains elusive. Procrastination becomes a familiar foe, as the allure of instant gratification trumps the foresight of future consequences.

In the realm of social interaction, ADHD can present its own set of challenges. Students with ADHD may struggle with impulsivity, blurting out responses without waiting their turn or interrupting others mid-conversation. These behaviours, often misconstrued as rudeness or lack of respect, can strain relationships with peers and professors alike, leading to feelings of isolation and alienation.

Despite these obstacles, it's crucial to recognise that students with ADHD possess a unique set of strengths that often go overlooked. Their boundless creativity, penchant for out-of-the-box thinking, and hyperfocus on topics of interest can be powerful assets in the academic arena when harnessed effectively.

Addressing the needs of students with ADHD in academic settings requires a multifaceted approach. First and foremost, it demands a paradigm shift in how we conceptualise and accommodate neurodiversity within educational institutions. Rather than viewing ADHD as a deficit to be remedied, it's imperative to adopt a strengths-based approach that celebrates the diverse cognitive profiles of all students.

Practical accommodations such as extended time for exams, preferential seating to minimise distractions, and access to assistive technologies can level the playing field for students with ADHD, allowing them to demonstrate their true potential. Moreover, fostering a supportive and inclusive learning environment where students feel empowered to advocate for their needs without fear of stigma or judgment is paramount.

Educators play a pivotal role in championing the academic success of students with ADHD by employing flexible teaching strategies that accommodate different learning styles and providing personalised feedback and encouragement. By cultivating a culture of empathy, understanding, and acceptance, academic institutions can pave the way for students with ADHD to thrive academically and beyond.

In the face of adversity, students with ADHD demonstrate remarkable resilience and tenacity, navigating the tumultuous waters of academia with unwavering determination. They are not defined by their challenges but rather by their ability to overcome them, transforming obstacles into opportunities for growth and self-discovery. As we strive to create a more inclusive and equitable educational landscape, let us not forget to amplify the voices of those whose struggles have long been marginalised, for it is in embracing diversity that we unlock the full potential of our collective humanity. the academic terrain is often a labyrinth of challenges for many students, but for those grappling with attention deficit hyperactivity disorder (ADHD), the journey can feel like traversing through a dense fog. ADHD, characterised by difficulties in concentration, impulse control, and hyperactivity, casts its shadow over every facet of life, including academia. For these students, the classroom becomes a battleground where traditional learning structures often clash with their unique cognitive makeup, leaving them feeling overwhelmed and misunderstood.

Getting Support from Educators and Accommodations and Learn to Excel in School

Navigating the educational landscape with attention deficit hyperactivity disorder (ADHD) can be akin to traversing a minefield. Yet, armed with the right support and accommodations, students with ADHD can not only survive but also thrive academically. The journey begins with fostering open communication and understanding between educators and students, laying the groundwork for a collaborative approach to learning.

For students with ADHD, securing support from educators is paramount to their success. This begins with self-advocacy—empowering students to articulate their needs and challenges in a constructive manner. By fostering a culture of openness and acceptance, educators can create a safe space where students feel comfortable expressing their concerns without fear of judgment or stigma.

Once the lines of communication are established, educators can work hand in hand with students to identify appropriate accommodations tailored to their individual needs. These accommodations may include extended time for assignments and exams, preferential seating to minimise distractions, access to assistive technologies, and breaks to help manage attention and energy levels.

Moreover, educators can employ flexible teaching strategies that cater to the diverse learning styles of students with ADHD. Breaking down complex concepts into bite-sized chunks, incorporating visual aids and interactive activities, and providing frequent feedback and reinforcement can enhance engagement and comprehension.

Beyond accommodations, fostering a supportive and inclusive learning environment is essential for students with ADHD to thrive. This involves cultivating a sense of belonging and community within the classroom, where students feel valued and accepted for who they are. Peer support groups and mentorship programs can also provide invaluable resources for students to connect with others who share similar experiences.

In addition to external support, students with ADHD can also develop their own strategies for success. This may involve implementing effective time management techniques, breaking tasks down into manageable steps, and utilising tools such as planners and organisers to stay organised. Building routines and establishing clear goals can also help students stay on track and maintain focus amidst the chaos of academic life.

It's important to recognise that success looks different for every student, and progress should be celebrated in all its forms. By fostering a growth mindset and emphasising effort over outcomes, educators can instil resilience and perseverance in students with ADHD, empowering them to overcome obstacles and reach their full potential.

In the end, excelling in school with ADHD is not just about overcoming challenges—it's about embracing one's unique strengths and finding creative ways to thrive in an environment that may not always cater to their needs. With the right support, accommodations, and mindset, students with ADHD can unlock a world of possibilities and achieve greatness beyond measure.

6. Managing Relationships:

- Struggling with maintaining friendships and romantic relationships.

- Working on communication skills and boundaries to foster healthy connections.

Struggling With Maintaining Friendships and Romantic Relationships

Navigating the intricate dance of human connection is a feat in itself, but for individuals grappling with attention deficit hyperactivity disorder (ADHD), maintaining friendships and romantic relationships can feel like traversing a labyrinth with no map. The unique cognitive profile associated with ADHD, characterised by difficulties in attention, impulse control, and emotional regulation, casts its shadow over every aspect of social interaction, presenting a myriad of challenges that can strain even the strongest of bonds.

For many individuals with ADHD, the constant whirlwind of thoughts and distractions makes it arduous to sustain meaningful connections with others. Conversations become a delicate balancing act, as their minds flit from one topic to another like a butterfly in a garden of ideas, leaving friends and romantic partners feeling sidelined or unheard. Consequently, the depth of intimacy and connection that others may take for granted remains elusive, leaving individuals with ADHD feeling isolated and misunderstood.

Moreover, the impulsivity that often accompanies ADHD can wreak havoc on social interactions, leading to misunderstandings and hurt feelings. Blurting out inappropriate comments without thinking, interrupting others mid-conversation, or acting on fleeting emotions without considering the consequences can strain relationships and erode trust over time. What may seem like spontaneity to some may come across as recklessness to others, further complicating the delicate dance of social interaction.

In romantic relationships, the challenges posed by ADHD can be particularly pronounced. The hyperfocus that individuals with ADHD may exhibit on their partner during the honeymoon phase of a relationship can quickly fade as the novelty wears off, leaving partners feeling neglected or abandoned. Similarly, the impulsivity and emotional volatility associated with ADHD can fuel conflict and tension within the relationship, as partners struggle to navigate the unpredictable terrain of their loved one's emotions.

Despite these challenges, it's important to recognise that individuals with ADHD possess a wealth of strengths that can enrich their relationships when harnessed effectively. Their boundless creativity, spontaneity, and zest for life can infuse relationships with energy and excitement, creating moments of joy and spontaneity that are truly unforgettable.

Building and maintaining friendships and romantic relationships with ADHD requires a multifaceted approach that addresses the unique needs and challenges of each individual. This may involve developing effective communication skills, setting boundaries, and cultivating self-awareness and empathy for both one and others. Seeking therapy or counselling can also provide invaluable support and guidance for navigating the complexities of interpersonal relationships.

Ultimately, the key to thriving in relationships with ADHD lies in embracing one's authentic self and finding partners and friends who accept and appreciate them for who they are. By fostering understanding, patience, and acceptance, individuals with ADHD can cultivate deep and meaningful connections that withstand the test of time, enriching their lives and the lives of those around them in ways they never thought possible.

Working On Communication Skills and Boundaries to Foster Health Connections

Navigating human connection is a delicate art, one that often proves particularly challenging for individuals grappling with attention deficit hyperactivity disorder (ADHD). Amidst the whirlwind of thoughts and emotions that characterise ADHD, maintaining healthy friendships and romantic relationships can feel like trying to navigate a maze blindfolded. However, with a mindful approach focused on communication skills and boundaries, individuals with ADHD can forge meaningful connections that withstand the test of time.

At the heart of fostering healthy connections lies the cornerstone of effective communication. For individuals with ADHD, communication can be a double-edged sword, both a source of frustration and a catalyst for growth. Learning to express thoughts and emotions clearly and assertively, while also actively listening to others with empathy and understanding, lays the groundwork for building strong and resilient relationships.

One of the key challenges individuals with ADHD face in communication is managing impulsivity and hyperactivity. The urge to interject or speak without fully considering the consequences can lead to misunderstandings and conflict. By practicing mindfulness and self-awareness, individuals can learn to pause and reflect before responding, allowing for more thoughtful and deliberate communication.

Additionally, honing skills in nonverbal communication—such as maintaining eye contact, interpreting body language, and regulating facial expressions—can help bridge the gap between intention and interpretation, fostering deeper connections with others.

Boundaries serve as the scaffolding upon which healthy relationships are built, providing a framework for mutual respect and autonomy. For individuals with ADHD, maintaining boundaries can be particularly challenging, as impulsivity and difficulty with time management may lead to overcommitment or boundary violations.

Learning to set clear and consistent boundaries, as well as respecting the boundaries of others, is essential for fostering healthy connections. This may involve communicating personal needs and limitations openly and assertively, as well as recognising when it's necessary to say no or renegotiate existing boundaries.

Furthermore, establishing routines and structures can help individuals with ADHD better manage their time and energy, reducing the likelihood of overextending themselves or neglecting self-care in favour of social obligations.

In romantic relationships, communication and boundaries take on added significance, serving as the bedrock of intimacy and trust. Couples counselling or therapy can provide a safe space for partners to explore and address issues related to ADHD, fostering greater understanding and empathy between both parties.

Ultimately, fostering healthy connections with ADHD requires a combination of self-awareness, mindfulness, and a willingness to learn and grow. By honing communication skills, setting clear boundaries, and prioritising self-care, individuals with ADHD can cultivate meaningful and fulfilling relationships that enrich their lives and those of their loved ones.

7. Career Exploration:

- Entering the workforce and encountering difficulties in finding and maintaining employment.

- With career counselling and workplace accommodations, discovering fulfilling career paths that align with the strengths.

Entering The Workforce and Encountering Difficulties in Finding and Maintaining Employment

Entering the workforce marks a significant milestone in one's journey toward independence and self-sufficiency. However, for individuals grappling with attention deficit hyperactivity disorder (ADHD), the transition from academia to the professional realm can be fraught with unique challenges and hurdles. From navigating job interviews to managing workplace expectations, finding and maintaining employment with ADHD requires resilience, adaptation, and a supportive network of resources.

One of the primary obstacles individuals with ADHD encounter when seeking employment is the daunting task of job hunting itself. The traditional job application process, with its emphasis on meticulous attention to detail and sustained focus, can feel like a Herculean feat for those grappling with ADHD symptoms such as impulsivity, distractibility, and difficulty with organisation.

Moreover, job interviews—a staple of the hiring process —can be particularly daunting for individuals with ADHD. The pressure to articulate skills and qualifications coherently while under scrutiny can exacerbate feelings of anxiety and self-doubt. Strategies such as practicing mock interviews, seeking support from career counsellors or mentors, and disclosing ADHD-related accommodations to potential employers can help level the playing field and increase the likelihood of success.

Once employed, individuals with ADHD may encounter difficulties in navigating the demands of the workplace. Challenges such as maintaining focus on tasks, meeting deadlines, and managing time effectively can undermine job performance and erode self-confidence. Moreover, workplace environments characterised by noise, distractions, and constant interruptions can exacerbate symptoms and impede productivity.

In addition to the practical challenges of the workplace, individuals with ADHD may also face stigma and misconceptions surrounding their condition. Misunderstandings about ADHD—such as viewing it as a character flaw or a lack of willpower—can lead to discrimination and bias in hiring and promotion decisions. Educating employers and coworkers about ADHD, advocating for workplace accommodations, and seeking support from disability services or employee assistance programs can help mitigate these barriers and foster a more inclusive and supportive work environment.

Despite these challenges, it's important to recognise that individuals with ADHD possess a unique set of strengths and talents that can be invaluable assets in the workplace. Creativity, resilience, adaptability, and a knack for thinking outside the box are just a few of the qualities that individuals with ADHD bring to the table. By leveraging these strengths, seeking out supportive environments, and advocating for their needs, individuals with ADHD can carve out fulfilling and successful careers that allow them to thrive professionally and personally.

In conclusion, finding and maintaining employment with ADHD may present its share of obstacles, but with perseverance, self-awareness, and a proactive approach, individuals with ADHD can overcome these challenges and achieve their career goals. By embracing their unique strengths and seeking out supportive resources, individuals with ADHD can unlock their full potential and make meaningful contributions to the workforce and society at large.

Career Counselling and Workplace Accommodations, Discovering Fulfilling Career Paths That Align with the Strengths

Navigating the professional landscape with attention deficit hyperactivity disorder (ADHD) can feel like embarking on a labyrinthine journey, fraught with uncertainty and challenges. However, with the guidance of career counselling and the implementation of workplace accommodations, individuals with ADHD can chart a course toward fulfilling career paths that not only capitalise on their strengths but also align with their passions and aspirations.

Career counselling serves as a beacon of light in the fog of career indecision, providing individuals with ADHD the tools and resources they need to explore their interests, values, and skills. Through assessments, self-reflection exercises, and one-on-one sessions with experienced counsellors, individuals can gain clarity about their career goals and identify potential paths that resonate with their unique strengths and talents.

One of the key benefits of career counselling for individuals with ADHD is its focus on holistic assessment and personalised guidance. Rather than adhering to a one-size-fits-all approach, career counsellors work collaboratively with clients to tailor strategies and interventions that address their specific needs and challenges. This may involve exploring alternative career paths that prioritise creativity, flexibility, and autonomy, or identifying accommodations that can mitigate the impact of ADHD symptoms in the workplace.

Moreover, career counselling can help individuals with ADHD develop essential skills for career success, such as time management, organisation, and effective communication. By equipping clients with practical tools and strategies to navigate the demands of the professional world, career counsellors empower individuals to overcome obstacles and capitalise on their strengths.

In addition to career counselling, workplace accommodations play a crucial role in supporting individuals with ADHD in their career journeys. Accommodations such as flexible work hours, remote work options, and assistive technologies can help individuals manage symptoms such as impulsivity, distractibility, and difficulty with time management. Moreover, accommodations that foster a supportive and inclusive work environment, such as clear communication and feedback, structured routines, and opportunities for professional development, can enhance job satisfaction and retention for individuals with ADHD.

By leveraging the insights gained through career counselling and the support provided by workplace accommodations, individuals with ADHD can discover fulfilling career paths that harness their unique strengths and talents. Whether pursuing creative endeavours, entrepreneurial ventures, or traditional professions, individuals with ADHD have the potential to make meaningful contributions to their chosen fields and thrive in their careers.

Career counselling and workplace accommodations serve as invaluable resources for individuals with ADHD seeking to navigate the complexities of the professional world. By embracing their strengths, advocating for their needs, and leveraging the support of counsellors and employers, individuals with ADHD can unlock their full potential and embark on fulfilling career paths that align with their passions and aspirations.

8. Overcoming Obstacles:

- Despite progress, facing setbacks and obstacles along the way.

- Experiencing periods of frustration and self-doubt but persevere through resilience and determination.

Despite Progress, Facing Setbacks and Obstacles Along the Way

Despite the strides made in understanding and accommodating attention deficit hyperactivity disorder (ADHD), individuals on this journey often find themselves confronting setbacks and obstacles that can feel like stumbling blocks on the path to success. The road to managing ADHD is rarely linear, marked instead by peaks and valleys, triumphs and tribulations. Yet, within these setbacks lie opportunities for growth, resilience, and self-discovery.

One of the most formidable obstacles individuals with ADHD face is the pervasive stigma and misconceptions surrounding the disorder. Despite increased awareness and advocacy efforts, ADHD continues to be shrouded in misunderstanding, with many misconstruing it as a mere lack of discipline or willpower. This stigma can manifest in various spheres of life, from education to employment, often leading to feelings of shame, self-doubt, and isolation.

Moreover, the symptoms of ADHD themselves can pose significant challenges in daily life. Difficulties with attention, impulsivity, and hyperactivity can impede academic performance, disrupt relationships, and hinder professional success. Individuals with ADHD may struggle to stay organised, manage time effectively, and regulate their emotions, leading to frustration and feelings of inadequacy.

In the realm of education, students with ADHD may encounter barriers to learning, such as difficulty focusing on class, keeping up with assignments, and navigating the demands of standardised testing. Despite their best efforts, setbacks such as poor grades, academic probation, or even disciplinary action may occur, further exacerbating feelings of frustration and discouragement.

Similarly, in the workforce, individuals with ADHD may face challenges in finding and maintaining employment, as well as advancing in their careers. Workplace environments characterised by noise, distractions, and rigid structures can exacerbate ADHD symptoms and impede productivity. Moreover, stigma and misconceptions surrounding ADHD may lead to discrimination and bias in hiring and promotion decisions, limiting opportunities for professional growth and advancement.

Despite these setbacks and obstacles, it's important to recognise that progress is possible. With the right support, resources, and mindset, individuals with ADHD can overcome challenges and achieve their goals. This may involve seeking out accommodations, such as therapy, medication, or assistive technologies, that can help mitigate symptoms and enhance functioning. Building a strong support network of friends, family, and professionals who understand and validate their experiences can also provide invaluable support on the journey.

Furthermore, reframing setbacks as opportunities for learning and growth can help individuals with ADHD develop resilience and perseverance in the face of adversity. By embracing their unique strengths, talents, and perspectives, individuals with ADHD can harness their full potential and make meaningful contributions to their communities and the world at large.

Facing setbacks and obstacles along the journey with ADHD is an inevitable part of the process. However, by cultivating resilience, seeking support, and embracing opportunities for growth, individuals with ADHD can navigate these challenges and forge a path toward a brighter, more fulfilling future.

Experiencing Periods of Frustration and Self Doubt but Persevere Through Resilience and Determination

Living with Attention Deficit Hyperactivity Disorder (ADHD) is often a rollercoaster ride of highs and lows, marked by periods of frustration and self-doubt. The constant struggle to stay focused, organised, and on task can take its toll, leading to moments of despair and uncertainty. Yet, within the depths of these challenges lies a reservoir of resilience and determination that enables individuals with ADHD to persevere in the face of adversity.

Frustration becomes a familiar companion for those navigating life with ADHD. Tasks that seem simple to others—a mundane chore, a routine assignment—can morph into insurmountable obstacles, leaving individuals feeling overwhelmed and defeated. The inability to stay on track, coupled with a relentless inner critic, fuels a cycle of frustration that threatens to engulf even the most resilient spirit.

Self-doubt lurks in the shadows, whispering tales of inadequacy and failure. Despite their best efforts, individuals with ADHD may find themselves questioning their abilities, their worth, and their place in the world. The constant barrage of setbacks and challenges can erode confidence, leaving behind a hollow shell of doubt and insecurity.

Yet, amidst the chaos and turmoil, a flicker of resilience emerges—a beacon of hope in the darkness. Resilience is the quiet strength that resides within each individual with ADHD, a steadfast resolve to persevere in the face of adversity. It is the courage to pick oneself up after every fall, to dust off the ashes of defeat, and to forge ahead with unwavering determination.

Determination becomes the driving force that propels individuals with ADHD forward on their journey. It is the fierce determination to defy the odds, to challenge the status quo, and to carve out a path of their own making. Despite the naysayers and the doubters, individuals with ADHD cling to their dreams with an unyielding tenacity, refusing to let their struggles define them.

Through the trials and tribulations, individuals with ADHD discover their inner strength—the resilience to weather life's storms and emerge stronger on the other side. They learn to harness their unique gifts and talents, transforming adversity into opportunity, and self-doubt into self-discovery. With each setback overcome, they grow more resilient, more determined, and more capable of facing whatever challenges lie ahead.

Moreover, they draw strength from their support networks —friends, family, mentors, and professionals who stand by their side, offering encouragement, guidance, and unwavering belief in their potential. Together, they weather the storms of uncertainty, celebrating victories both big and small and lifting each other up when the weight of the world feels too heavy to bear alone.

In the end, the journey with ADHD is not defined by the struggles encountered along the way, but by the resilience and determination with which they are met. It is a testament to the indomitable spirit of the human heart, a reminder that within every setback lies the seed of opportunity, and within every challenge, the potential for growth. As individuals with ADHD persevere through resilience and determination, they inspire others to do the same, forging a path toward a brighter, more hopeful future for all.

9. Building a Support Network:

- Finding support and camaraderie in ADHD support groups and communities.

- Forming meaningful connections with others who share similar experiences and challenges.

Finding Support and Camaraderie in ADHD Support Groups and Communities

Navigating life with attention deficit hyperactivity disorder (ADHD) can often feel like embarking on a solitary journey through uncharted territory, with challenges and obstacles lurking around every corner. However, within the vast landscape of the ADHD community lies a beacon of hope— a network of support groups and communities that offer solace, understanding, and camaraderie to those who walk this path.

For many individuals with ADHD, the journey begins with a sense of isolation—a feeling of being different, misunderstood, or out of sync with the world around them. Yet, upon discovering the rich tapestry of ADHD support groups and communities, they find a sanctuary— a place where their experiences are not only validated but celebrated.

In these spaces, individuals with ADHD come together to share their stories, exchange insights, and offer encouragement to one another. Here, they find a sense of belonging—a tribe of kindred spirits who understand the unique challenges they face and offer unwavering support and camaraderie in return.

Support groups provide a safe space for individuals with ADHD to express themselves openly and honestly, free from judgment or stigma. Whether in-person or online, these gatherings offer a platform for individuals to share their triumphs and tribulations, seek advice and guidance, and form meaningful connections with others who share similar experiences.

Moreover, support groups serve as a valuable source of information and resources for individuals seeking to better understand and manage their ADHD. Through workshops, seminars, and guest speakers, participants gain practical strategies and coping mechanisms for navigating the challenges of daily life—from managing time and organisation to improving communication and self-care.

In addition to support groups, online communities play a vital role in fostering connection and camaraderie among individuals with ADHD. Through forums, social media groups, and virtual meetups, individuals can connect with peers from around the world, transcending geographic boundaries to find solidarity in shared experiences.

Within these communities, individuals with ADHD find not only support but also empowerment— the knowledge that they are not defined by their diagnosis but rather by their resilience, strength, and tenacity. Together, they celebrate each other's successes, offer a shoulder to lean on in times of need, and champion one another as they navigate the highs and lows of life with ADHD.

Finding support and camaraderie in ADHD support groups and communities is a beacon of hope for individuals navigating the complexities of life with ADHD. Through shared experiences, mutual understanding, and unwavering support, individuals with ADHD find solace, validation, and empowerment in the knowledge that they are not alone on this journey. Together, they forge bonds that transcend diagnosis, building a community founded on compassion, empathy, and the shared quest for a brighter tomorrow.

Forming Meaningful Connections with Others Who Share Similar Experiences and Challenges

Forming meaningful connections with others who share similar experiences and challenges with attention deficit hyperactivity disorder (ADHD) is akin to discovering a hidden treasure—a priceless gift that enriches the journey of self-discovery and growth. In a world where individuals with ADHD often feel misunderstood or isolated, finding kinship with kindred spirits who walk a similar path can be a source of solace, validation, and empowerment.

One of the most profound aspects of connecting with others who have ADHD is the instant recognition of shared experiences. There is an unspoken understanding —an invisible thread that binds individuals together in a tapestry of empathy and understanding. Whether swapping stories of forgetfulness, impulsivity, or hyperfocus, there is a sense of relief in knowing that one is not alone in grappling with the quirks and nuances of ADHD.

Moreover, connecting with others who have ADHD provides a unique opportunity for validation and affirmation. In a world where ADHD is often misunderstood or stigmatised, finding acceptance and understanding among peers who share similar struggles can be transformative. It offers a sense of belonging—a reminder that one's experiences are valid and worthy of acknowledgment.

Beyond validation, forming connections with others who have ADHD offers a source of practical support and guidance. Whether seeking advice on managing symptoms, navigating challenges in school or the workplace, or finding resources and accommodations, peers can offer valuable insights and strategies based on their own experiences. Through shared wisdom and collective knowledge, individuals with ADHD can learn from one another and empower each other to thrive.

Furthermore, connecting with others who have ADHD fosters a sense of community—a shared bond that transcends diagnosis. In these connections, individuals find companionship, friendship, and camaraderie. They celebrate each other's successes, offer support in times of need, and champion one another's growth and resilience.

In addition to offering support and understanding, forming connections with others who have ADHD can also be a source of inspiration and motivation. Witnessing the accomplishments and achievements of peers who have overcome similar challenges can instil hope and confidence in one's own abilities. It serves as a reminder that ADHD is not a limitation but rather a unique lens through which to view the world—a lens that can illuminate new possibilities and pathways forward.

Forming meaningful connections with others who share similar experiences and challenges with ADHD is a powerful catalyst for growth, healing, and transformation. Through empathy, validation, and support, individuals with ADHD find solace in knowing that they are not alone on their journey. Together, they forge bonds that transcend diagnosis, building a community founded on understanding, acceptance, and the shared pursuit of a brighter tomorrow.

10. Advocacy and Empowerment:

- Inspired by the journey, becoming an advocate for ADHD awareness and acceptance.

- Sharing your story publicly, advocating for improved resources and support for individuals with ADHD.

Inspired By the Journey, Becoming and Advocate for ADHD Awareness and Acceptance

Embarking on the journey with attention deficit hyperactivity disorder (ADHD) is not merely a solitary voyage—it is an odyssey of self-discovery, resilience, and empowerment. Along this winding path, individuals with ADHD often find themselves transformed—not only by the challenges they face but by the strength and courage they discover within themselves. Inspired by their own journey, many individuals with ADHD become passionate advocates for ADHD awareness and acceptance, championing the cause with unwavering determination and fervour.

For many, the decision to become an advocate arises from a deeply personal place—a desire to shatter the silence and stigma surrounding ADHD and to shine a light on the lived experiences of those affected by the disorder. Drawing upon their own struggles and triumphs, individuals with ADHD become voices for change, speaking out against misconceptions and discrimination and advocating for greater understanding and support.

One of the most powerful tools in the advocate's arsenal is storytelling. Through sharing their own stories and experiences, individuals with ADHD offer a glimpse into the realities of living with the disorder, humanising the challenges and triumphs that accompany it. By putting a face to ADHD and sharing their journey with authenticity and vulnerability, advocates inspire empathy, compassion, and solidarity among others.

Moreover, advocates for ADHD awareness and acceptance work tirelessly to dispel myths and misconceptions surrounding the disorder. They educate the public about the neurobiological basis of ADHD, challenging stereotypes and stigma with evidence-based information and research. By raising awareness and promoting understanding, advocates pave the way for greater acceptance and support for individuals with ADHD in all aspects of life.

In addition to raising awareness, advocates for ADHD strive to improve access to resources and support for individuals affected by the disorder. They work collaboratively with policymakers, healthcare professionals, educators, and community organisations to advocate for policies and initiatives that address the needs of individuals with ADHD—from improving access to diagnosis and treatment to promoting accommodations and support services in schools and workplaces.

Furthermore, advocates for ADHD empowerment and acceptance promote self-advocacy and resilience among individuals with ADHD, empowering them to embrace their strengths, advocate for their needs, and pursue their goals with confidence and determination. By fostering a culture of acceptance and support, advocates create a ripple effect of positive change, transforming communities and institutions to better serve the needs of individuals with ADHD.

Inspired by their own journey, individuals with ADHD become passionate advocates for ADHD awareness and acceptance, working tirelessly to shatter stigma, promote

understanding, and empower others to thrive. Through storytelling, education, and advocacy, they inspire empathy, compassion, and solidarity, creating a more inclusive and supportive world for all individuals affected by ADHD.

Sharing Your Story Publicly, Advocating for Improved Resources and Support for Individuals With Sharing your story publicly and advocating for improved resources and support for individuals with attention deficit hyperactivity disorder (ADHD) is a courageous act of empowerment—a declaration that your experiences matter, your voice deserves to be heard, and your journey has the power to inspire change. For many individuals with ADHD, the decision to share their story publicly is deeply personal, born from a desire to break the silence and stigma surrounding the disorder. It is a testament to their resilience and strength—a bold declaration that they refuse to be defined by their challenges but instead choose to embrace their experiences as sources of wisdom, compassion, and empathy. Through sharing their story, individuals with ADHD offer a window into the realities of living with the disorder, illuminating the triumphs and tribulations that accompany it. They provide a voice for the voiceless, a beacon of hope for those who feel lost or alone in their struggles. By speaking out with authenticity and vulnerability, they inspire others to find solace in their shared experiences and to embrace their own journeys with courage and grace. Moreover, sharing your story publicly serves as a powerful form of advocacy—a call to action to improve resources and support for individuals with ADHD. By shedding light on the challenges faced by those affected by the disorder, advocates catalyse change, igniting conversations and driving momentum for reform. Advocates for improved resources and support for individuals with ADHD work tirelessly to raise awareness and promote understanding of the disorder. They educate the public about the neurobiological basis of ADHD, dispelling myths and misconceptions with evidence-based information and research. By challenging stereotypes and stigma, they create a more inclusive and supportive environment for individuals with ADHD to thrive. In addition to raising awareness, advocates for improved resources and support for individuals with ADHD push for systemic change, advocating for policies and initiatives that address the needs of those affected by the disorder. They collaborate with policymakers, healthcare professionals, educators, and community organisations to develop and implement programs and services that promote early intervention, access to diagnosis and treatment, and accommodations and support in schools and workplaces. Furthermore, advocates for improved resources and support for individuals with ADHD empower individuals to become agents of change in their own lives. They encourage self-advocacy and resilience, equipping individuals with the tools and resources they need to navigate the challenges of living with ADHD and to pursue their goals with confidence and determination. Sharing your story publicly and advocating for improved resources and support for individuals with ADHD is a powerful act of empowerment and advocacy. By speaking out with authenticity and vulnerability, individuals with ADHD inspire change, driving momentum for reform and creating a more inclusive and supportive world for all those affected by the disorder.

11. Finding Balance:

Striking a balance between managing their ADHD symptoms and embracing your true self.

Prioritising self-care, mindfulness, and healthy habits to maintain overall wellbeing.

Striking A Balance Between Managing Your ADHD
Symptoms and Embracing Your True Self

Striking a balance between managing attention deficit
hyperactivity disorder (ADHD) symptoms and embracing
one's true self is a delicate dance—a journey of self-
discovery, acceptance, and empowerment. For
individuals with ADHD, navigating this balance requires a
deep understanding of their strengths and challenges, as
well as a commitment to self-compassion, resilience, and
growth.

At the heart of this balance lies the recognition that ADHD
is not a flaw to be fixed but rather a unique aspect of
one's identity—a lens through which to view the world.
Embracing one's true self means accepting all facets of
who you are, including the quirks and idiosyncrasies that
come with ADHD. It means acknowledging that ADHD is
just one part of the intricate tapestry of your identity, not
the sum total of who you are as a person.

Managing ADHD symptoms involves a multifaceted
approach that encompasses both practical strategies and
emotional resilience. It means learning to navigate the
challenges of impulsivity, distractibility, and hyperactivity
with grace and compassion. It means developing coping
mechanisms and strategies for managing time,
organisation, and focus, while also recognising that
perfection is an unrealistic standard and that setbacks
are a natural part of the journey.

Moreover, managing ADHD symptoms involves seeking
out support and resources that can help you thrive. This

may involve therapy, medication, or other treatments that can help mitigate symptoms and enhance functioning. It may also involve building a support network of friends, family, and professionals who understand and validate your experiences, offering encouragement, guidance, and empathy along the way.

However, managing ADHD symptoms should not come at the expense of embracing your true self. It's essential to remember that you are more than your diagnosis—that you are a complex, multifaceted individual with hopes, dreams, and passions that transcend ADHD. Embracing your true self means honouring your strengths, talents, and interests, while also acknowledging your vulnerabilities and areas for growth.

Finding balance between managing ADHD symptoms and embracing your true self requires self-awareness, mindfulness, and self-compassion. It means listening to your body and mind, honouring your needs, and setting boundaries that prioritise your well-being. It means recognising that self-care is not selfish but essential for maintaining equilibrium in a world that often feels overwhelming.

Ultimately, finding balance between managing ADHD symptoms and embracing your true self is an ongoing journey—one that requires patience, perseverance, and a willingness to learn and grow. It's about finding harmony between acceptance and action, between self-compassion and resilience. By embracing who you are, ADHD and all, you empower yourself to live authentically and fully, embracing the richness and complexity of the human experience.

Prioritising Self-care, Mindfulness, And Healthy Habits to Maintain Overall Well-being

Prioritising self-care, mindfulness, and healthy habits is not just a luxury—it's a necessity, especially for individuals navigating the complexities of life with attention deficit hyperactivity disorder (ADHD). In a world that often feels chaotic and overwhelming, carving out time for self-care becomes an essential lifeline—a sanctuary of calm amidst the storm.

At the heart of prioritising self-care with ADHD lies the recognition that mental and emotional wellbeing are just as important as physical health. Self-care isn't selfish— it's an act of self-preservation, a commitment to nurturing your mind, body, and spirit so that you can show up fully in all areas of your life.

One of the cornerstones of self-care for individuals with ADHD is mindfulness—the practice of being present in the moment, without judgment or distraction. Mindfulness allows individuals to cultivate a sense of calm and clarity amidst the whirlwind of thoughts and emotions that characterise ADHD. By bringing attention to the present moment through practices such as meditation, deep breathing, or mindful movement, individuals with ADHD can quiet the noise of the mind and find a sense of peace within themselves.

In addition to mindfulness, prioritising self-care with ADHD involves cultivating healthy habits that support overall well-being. This may include regular exercise, balanced nutrition, adequate sleep, and stress management techniques. Engaging in physical activity not only boosts mood and energy levels but also helps to regulate dopamine levels in the brain—a neurotransmitter that plays a key role in ADHD. Similarly, eating a balanced diet rich in nutrients can help stabilise blood sugar levels and improve focus and concentration. Prioritising sleep is also crucial, as adequate rest allows the brain to recharge and replenish, enhancing cognitive function and mood stability.

Furthermore, managing stress and overwhelm is essential for maintaining overall well-being with ADHD. This may involve incorporating relaxation techniques such as yoga, tai chi, or progressive muscle relaxation into your daily routine. It may also involve setting boundaries, learning to say no to excessive commitments, and seeking support from friends, family, or mental health professionals when needed.

Self-care with ADHD is not a one-size-fits-all approach— it's about finding what works best for you and making it a priority in your life. It's about listening to your body and mind, honouring your needs, and setting boundaries that prioritise your well-being. It's about recognising that self-care is not selfish but essential for managing ADHD symptoms and thriving in all areas of your life.

Prioritising self-care, mindfulness, and healthy habits is a vital component of managing overall well-being with ADHD. By nurturing your mind, body, and spirit, you empower yourself to navigate the challenges of ADHD with resilience, grace, and strength. Remember, you are worthy of care and compassion—so prioritise yourself, because you deserve it.

Action and Growth:

- Reflecting on the journey of coping with ADHD and the lessons learned along the way.

 - Celebrating the achievements and acknowledge the progress made in embracing your identity.

Reflecting On the Journey of Coping with ADHD And the
Lessons Learned Along the Way

Reflecting on the journey of coping with attention deficit
hyperactivity disorder (ADHD) is akin to gazing into a
mirror—a journey of self-discovery, growth, and
transformation. Along this winding path, individuals with
ADHD navigate a landscape marked by triumphs and
tribulations, setbacks and successes, yet within the
depths of their experiences lie invaluable lessons that
illuminate the way forward.

One of the most profound lessons learned on the journey
with ADHD is the power of selfawareness. Through
introspection and reflection, individuals with ADHD gain
insight into their unique strengths and challenges,
learning to recognise patterns, triggers, and coping
mechanisms that shape their experiences. By cultivating
self-awareness, they empower themselves to navigate
the complexities of living with ADHD with greater clarity
and resilience.

Moreover, the journey with ADHD teaches the importance
of self-compassion—a gentle reminder that perfection is
an illusion and that setbacks are a natural part of the
process. Individuals with ADHD learn to embrace their
imperfections, treating themselves with kindness and
understanding in moments of frustration and self-doubt.
Through self-compassion, they cultivate resilience and
inner strength, allowing them to weather the storms of
uncertainty with grace and dignity.

Another crucial lesson learned on the journey with ADHD is the power of community and connection. Whether through support groups, online communities, or personal relationships, individuals with ADHD find solace and solidarity in connecting with others who share similar experiences. Through shared stories and shared struggles, they find validation, empathy, and understanding, fostering a sense of belonging that transcends diagnosis.

Furthermore, the journey with ADHD teaches the importance of resilience and perseverance. Despite the challenges and obstacles encountered along the way, individuals with ADHD learn to harness their inner strength and determination, refusing to be defined by their struggles. Through resilience, they transform setbacks into opportunities for growth, using adversity as a catalyst for positive change and personal development.

Additionally, the journey with ADHD teaches the importance of self-care and healthy habits. Individuals with ADHD learn to prioritise their well-being, incorporating mindfulness, exercise, and relaxation techniques into their daily routine. By nurturing their physical, mental, and emotional health, they cultivate a foundation of resilience and vitality that supports them on their journey toward greater well-being.

Reflecting on the journey of coping with ADHD is a profound and transformative experience—a journey of self-discovery, growth, and resilience. Through self-awareness, self-compassion, community, and resilience, individuals with ADHD navigate the complexities of living with the disorder with grace and dignity. And in the lessons learned along the way, they find wisdom, strength, and hope for the journey ahead.

Celebrating The Achievements and Acknowledge the
Process Made in Embracing Your Identity

Celebrating the achievements and acknowledging the
progress made in embracing one's identity with attention
deficit hyperactivity disorder (ADHD) is a testament to the
resilience, courage, and growth that define the journey
with this unique neurodevelopmental condition. From the
smallest victories to the most significant milestones, each
step forward is a triumph—a testament to the strength
and determination of individuals with ADHD to navigate
life with authenticity, purpose, and resilience.

For many individuals with ADHD, the journey toward self-
acceptance and empowerment is marked by a series of
pivotal moments—moments of clarity, insight, and
transformation that redefine their understanding of
themselves and their place in the world. It may be the
moment they recognise their strengths and talents as
gifts rather than limitations, or the moment they find the
courage to speak their truth and advocate for their needs
with confidence and conviction.

Each achievement, no matter how small, is cause for
celebration—a testament to the resilience and
perseverance that define the journey with ADHD.
Whether it's completing a project, mastering a new skill,

or simply getting through the day with grace and dignity, every accomplishment is a victory—a reminder of the progress made and the potential that lies within.

Moreover, celebrating achievements and acknowledging progress is an affirmation of the courage and resilience it takes to embrace one's identity with ADHD in a world that often misunderstands and stigmatises the disorder. It's a declaration that ADHD is not a limitation but a source of strength—an integral part of who you are that shapes your experiences, perspectives, and aspirations in profound ways.

In celebrating achievements and acknowledging progress, individuals with ADHD reclaim their narrative, rewriting the script of their lives with courage, resilience, and authenticity. They refuse to be defined by their struggles but instead choose to embrace their experiences as sources of wisdom, compassion, and empathy. They recognise that every obstacle overcome, every setback navigated, and every lesson learned is a testament to their strength and resilience—a reminder that they are capable of achieving greatness beyond measure.

Furthermore, celebrating achievements and acknowledging progress is a powerful form of selfcare—an affirmation of self-worth and validation that nourishes the soul and strengthens the spirit. It's a reminder that you are worthy of love, respect, and acceptance just as you are, and that your journey with ADHD is a testament to your courage, resilience, and determination to thrive.

Celebrating achievements and acknowledging progress in embracing one's identity with ADHD is a powerful affirmation of resilience, courage, and self-acceptance. It's a testament to the strength and determination of individuals with ADHD to navigate life with authenticity, purpose, and grace, and a reminder that every step forward is a triumph worth celebrating.